THE ULTIMATE YOGA GUIDE FOR BEGINNERS

Carol Hill

Table of Contents

INTRODUCTION
- *Understanding Yoga*
- *Benefits for Beginners*

GETTING STARTED WITH YOGA
- *Setting Up Your Practice Space*
- *Essential Yoga Equipment*

YOGA BASICS
- *Common Yoga Poses For Beginners*
- *Proper Breathing Techniques*

BUILDING A CONSISTENCE PRACTICE
- *Creating Your Yoga Routine*
- *Overcoming Common Challenges*

EXPLORING DIFFERENT YOGA STYLES
- *Overview of Popular Yoga Styles*
- *Finding the Style That Fits You*

INTEGRATING YOGA INTO DAILY LIFE
- *Bringing Yoga Off the Mat*
- *Sustaining a Lifelong Yoga Habit*

CHAPTER 1
INTRODUCTION

1.1 Understanding yoga:

Yoga is a holistic discipline that originated in ancient India, encompassing a multifaceted approach to harmonizing the mind, body, and spirit. Rooted in various philosophical traditions, the word "yoga" is derived from Sanskrit, meaning union or yoke, signifying the integration of different aspects of one's existence.

1a. Philosophical Foundations:

- ***Patanjali's Yoga Sutras:*** *Central to classical yoga, these sutras outline the eightfold path, known as Ashtanga, which serves as a guide for ethical and spiritual living.*

- ***Yamas and Niyamas:*** *The first two limbs of Ashtanga, emphasizing ethical* principles (yamas) and self-discipline (niyamas).

1b. Asana (Physical Postures):

- ***Hatha Yoga****: Focuses on physical postures (asanas) and breath control (pranayama) to achieve balance and prepare the body for meditation.*

- ***Vinyasa, Iyengar, and Bikram Yoga:*** *Different styles emphasizing flow, precision, and heat, respectively.*

1c. Pranayama (Breath Control):

- ***Breathing Techniques:*** *Pranayama involves various breath control techniques aimed at improving respiratory function, increasing vitality, and calming the mind.*

1d. Meditation and Dhyana:

- **Mindfulness and Concentration:** Integral to yoga, meditation cultivates heightened awareness, focus, and a deep sense of inner calm.
- **Transcendental Meditation and Zen Yoga:** Different traditions focusing on achieving states of transcendence and enlightenment.

1e. Mantra and Chanting:

- **Sacred Sounds:** The repetition of specific sounds or words (mantras) and chanting contribute to mental clarity, spiritual connection, and vibrational harmony.

1f. Yogic Diet and Lifestyle:

- **Sattvic Diet:** Emphasizes purity and balance, incorporating foods that promote clarity and vitality.
- **Aparigraha(Non-Attachment):** Encourages a minimalist lifestyle,

fostering detachment from material possessions.

1g. Mind-Body Connection:

- ***Yoga as Therapy:*** *Recognized for its therapeutic benefits, yoga is often used to alleviate physical ailments, manage stress, and enhance overall well-being.*
- ***Neuroscience and Yoga:*** *Research explores the impact of yoga on the brain, showing positive effects on cognitive function and emotional regulation.*

1h. Community and Sangha:

- ***Group Practice****: Many practitioners engage in communal yoga classes, creating a supportive environment for growth and shared experiences.*
- ***Global Yoga Community:*** *Yoga has transcended cultural boundaries, becoming worldwide phenomenon with diverse interpretations and practices.*

In essence, yoga serves as a comprehensive system fostering self-awareness, physical health, and spiritual growth. Its transformative potential extends beyond the mat, influencing daily life, relationships, and one's connection to the broader universe.

2.2 Benefits for Beginners:

Yoga is important for various reasons, encompassing physical, mental, and emotional well-being.

2a. Physical Health:

- ***Flexibility:*** *Yoga involves a wide range of poses that enhance flexibility, promoting better joint health and reducing the risk of injuries.*

- ***Strength:*** *Many yoga poses require supporting your body weight, contributing to muscle strength and tone.*

- **Balance and Posture:** *Regular practice improves balance and posture, aiding in overall physical stability.*

2b. Mental well-being:

- **Stress Reduction:** *Mindful breathing and meditation in yoga help reduce stress by activating the relaxation response, lowering cortisol levels.*

- **Mood Enhancement:** *Yoga promotes the release of endorphins, fostering a positive mood and alleviating symptoms of anxiety and depression.*

- **Focus and concentration:** *Mindfulness practices in yoga improve cognitive function, enhancing concentration and attention span.*

2c. Emotional Balance:

- **Self-awareness:** *Yoga encourages self-reflection, fostering a deeper understanding of emotions and thought patterns.*

- **Emotional Resilience:** *The practice teaches coping mechanisms, helping individuals better manage challenging situations.*

2d. Holistic Wellness:

- **Breath Control (Pranayama):** *Controlled breathing exercises enhance respiratory function, reduce stress, and improve overall lung capacity.*

- **Mind-Body Connection:** *Yoga emphasizes the interconnectedness of mind and body, promoting holistic well-beinge.*

2e. Health Benefits:

- **Improved Circulation:** Yoga poses enhance blood flow, aiding in better circulation and cardiovascular health.
- **Lower Blood Pressure:** Regular practice has been linked to reduced blood pressure, contributing to heart health.

- **Enhanced Immunity:** The combination of physical movement, breathwork, and relaxation supports a robust immune system.

2f. Lifestyle:

- **Better Sleep:** Yoga's relaxation techniques can improve sleep quality and help manage insomnia.

- **Healthy Lifestyle Choices:** The mindfulness cultivated in yoga often extends to making healthier lifestyle choices, including diet and stress management.

2g. Community and Connection:

- ***Social Interaction:*** *Participating in group yoga classes fosters a sense of community and connection, positively impacting mental health.*

In essence, yoga is a holistic practice that addresses various facets of well-being, contributing to a healthier, more balanced lifestyle. Regular practice can lead to long-term positive effects on physical health, mental clarity, and emotional resilience.

CHAPTER 2
GETTING STARTED WITH YOGA

1.1 Setting Up Your Practice Space:

A yoga practice space is a dedicated area designed for the practice of yoga, fostering a calm and focused environment. Typically, it includes a flat and non-slippery surface, such as a yoga mat or a specialized flooring. The space should be clean and free from clutter, promoting a sense of tranquility.

- ***Choose a Quiet Space:*** *Select a quiet area with minimal distractions. This could be a spare room, a corner of a room, or any peaceful spot in your home.*

- ***Clear the Area:*** *Remove any clutter or obstacles to create a clean and safe practice space. This helps prevent accidents and allows for better focus.*

- ***Gather Essential Equipment:*** *Collect your yoga essentials, including a yoga* *mat, comfortable clothing, and any props you may need (blocks, straps, or cushions). These tools enhance your practice and provide support.*

- ***Set the Mood with Lighting:*** *Opt for natural light if possible. If not, use soft, diffused lighting to create a calming atmosphere. Consider adding candles or dimming the lights to enhance relaxation.*

- ***Ventilation:*** *Ensure good air circulation in the room. Proper ventilation is essential for a comfortable practice, especially if you'll be engaging in more vigorous sequences.*

- ***Choose Appropriate Music or Silence:*** *Some practitioners prefer a quiet space, while others enjoy soft, soothing music. Select what suits your preferences, creating an ambiance that enhances your experience.*

- ***Personalize with Decor:*** *Add personal touches like plants, inspirational quotes, or calming artwork. Creating a space that resonates with you makes it more inviting and conducive to regular practice.*

- ***Dress Comfortably:*** *Wear loose, comfortable clothing that allows for a full range of motion. This enhances your ability to perform yoga poses without restrictions.*

- ***Establish a Routine:*** *Set a consistent practice schedule. Whether it's morning or evening, having a routine helps make yoga a habit and part of your daily or weekly activities.*

- ***Mindful Preparation:*** *Before starting your session, take a few moments to center yourself. Practice mindfulness, deep breathing, or a short meditation to transition from daily activities to your yoga practice.*

- ***Follow a Beginner-Friendly Sequence:*** *Choose a beginner-friendly yoga sequence or follow an online video. Focus on foundational poses, proper alignment, and gradually progress as you become more comfortable.*

- ***Listen to Your Body:*** *Throughout your practice, pay attention to how your body feels. Respect your limits, avoid pushing yourself too hard, and make modifications as needed.*

- ***Cool Down and Relaxation:*** *Finish your practice with a cooldown, including gentle stretches and a brief relaxation period in Savasana (Corpse Pose). This helps integrate the benefits of your practice and promotes a sense of calm.*

Remember, the key is to create a space that encourages regular practice and aligns with your personal preferences and comfort.

Adjustments can be made over time as you deepen your yoga journey.

2.2 Essential Yoga Equipment:

Yoga equipment can enhance your practice by providing support, stability, and alignment. Props like mats, blocks, and straps help maintain proper form, prevent injury, and deepen stretches. While not essential, these tools can improve comfort and accessibility, making yoga more enjoyable and effective for practitioners of all levels.

- *Yoga Mat: Provides a comfortable and non-slip surface for practicing asanas (poses) and serves as a personal space for meditation.*

- *Yoga Blocks: Help in achieving proper alignment and provide support during certain poses, especially for beginners or individuals with limited flexibility.*

- ***Yoga Strap:*** *Assists in reaching and holding poses by extending your reach, making yoga accessible for various body types and levels of flexibility.*

- ***Yoga Blanket:*** *Offers padding and warmth during relaxation poses and meditation, ensuring comfort and aiding in maintaining focus.*

- ***Bolster:*** *Provides support for restorative poses, promoting relaxation and allowing the body to release tension.*

- ***Yoga Mat Cleaner:*** *Essential for maintaining hygiene by cleaning your mat regularly, preventing the buildup of bacteria and maintaining a clean practice space.*

- ***Meditation Cushion:*** *Helps maintain a comfortable seated posture during meditation, reducing strain on the knees and hips.*

- ***Yoga Towel:*** *Placed over the mat, it absorbs sweat and provides a slip-resistant surface, ensuring a secure grip during dynamic poses.*

- ***Yoga Bag:*** *Convenient for carrying and storing your yoga equipment, making it easy to transport your gear to and from the studio.*

- ***Yoga Wheel:*** *Aids in enhancing flexibility, balance, and strength by assisting in deepening stretches and opening up the chest and back.*

- ***Incense or Essential Oils:*** *Used to create a calming and pleasant atmosphere during practice, enhancing the overall yoga experience.*

- ***Yoga Bolster:*** *Supports various poses and provides comfort during relaxation, promoting proper alignment and relaxation.*

- ***Yoga Ball:*** *Helps improve core strength and stability through exercises and can be incorporated into yoga routines for added challenge.*

- ***Yoga Sandbag:*** *Placed on certain body parts during poses to deepen stretches and promote relaxation by applying gentle pressure.*

- ***Yoga Timer or App:*** *Helps manage the duration of poses and meditation sessions, ensuring a balanced and mindful practice.*

CHAPTER 3
YOGA BASICS

1.1 Common Yoga Poses For Beginners:

Yoga poses, or "asanas," encompass a variety of physical postures designed to promote strength, flexibility, balance, and relaxation. Some common poses include Downward Dog, Tree Pose, Warrior Pose, and Child's Pose. Each pose offers unique benefits for the body and mind.

- ***Mountain Pose (Tadasana):** Stand with feet together, arms by your sides, and weight evenly distributed. Engage muscles, lengthen the spine, and reach arms overhead, palms facing each other.*

- ***Downward-Facing Dog (Adho Mukha Svanasana):** Start on hands and knees, lift hips towards the ceiling, straighten legs, and press heels towards the floor. Keep arms and back straight, forming an inverted V shape.*

- ***Warrior I (Virabhadrasana I):*** *Step one foot back, bend the front knee, and extend arms overhead with palms facing each other. Square hips forward and maintain a strong, grounded stance.*

- ***Warrior II (Virabhadrasana II):*** *From Warrior I, open hips and shoulders to face the side. Extend arms parallel to the floor, aligning with shoulders. Front knee remains bent, tracking over the ankle.*

- ***Tree Pose (Vrksasana):*** *Stand on one leg, lift the opposite foot and place it on the inner thigh or calf (avoid the knee). Bring palms together in front of the chest or extend arms overhead.*

- ***Child's Pose (Balasana):*** *Kneel on the mat, sit back on heels, and extend arms forward, lowering the chest towards the floor. This restorative pose helps relax and stretch the back.*

- ***Cobra Pose (Bhujangasana):*** *Lie on your stomach, place hands beside the chest, and lift the upper body while keeping the pelvis on the floor. This strengthens the back and opens the chest.*

- ***Bridge Pose (Setu Bandhasana):*** *Lie on your back, bend knees, and place feet hip-width apart. Lift the hips towards the ceiling, interlace fingers beneath the back, and press shoulders into the mat.*

- ***Seated Forward Bend (Paschimottanasana):*** *Sit with legs extended, hinge at the hips, and reach towards the toes. Keep the back straight and engage the core. This stretches the spine and hamstrings.*

- ***Corpse Pose (Savasana):*** *Lie on your back, legs extended, and arms by your sides. Close your eyes, relax the entire body, and focus on your breath. It promotes deep relaxation and integration after a yoga session.*

2.2 Proper Breathing Techniques:

As explain form the previous chapters the breathing technique is the major technique in yoga.

Proper breathing, or pranayama, is crucial in yoga for several reasons, It enhances oxygen flow, increases energy levels, promotes relaxation, and helps focus the mind. Consistent practice of correct breathing techniques also improves lung capacity and supports overall well-being during yoga sessions.

- **Diaphragmatic Breathing (Dirga Pranayama):** This technique focuses on deep breaths, engaging the diaphragm to expand the lungs fully. Inhale deeply through the nose, allowing the abdomen to expand, then exhale completely, contracting the abdominal muscles. This promotes relaxation and reduces stress.

- ***Ujjayi Breath (Victorious Breath):*** *Ujjayi involves slightly constricting the back of the throat during both inhalation and exhalation, creating a soft, ocean-like sound. This technique enhances focus, warms the body, and encourages mindfulness during yoga practice.*

- ***Nadi Shodhana (Alternate Nostril Breathing):*** *Nadi Shodhana aims to balance the flow of energy in the body. Using the thumb and ring finger, alternate closing off one nostril while inhaling and exhaling through the other. This technique promotes a sense of calmness, concentration, and equilibrium.*

- ***Kapalabhati (Skull Shining Breath):*** *Kapalabhati involves forceful exhalations through the nose with passive inhalations. This rapid breathing technique cleanses the lungs, energizes the body, and enhances mental clarity. It* *is crucial to maintain a relaxed diaphragm during Kapalabhati.*

- **Bhramari Pranayama (Bee Breath):** *In Bhramari, the practitioner produces a humming sound during exhalation, resembling the buzzing of a bee. This technique helps release tension, soothes the nervous system, and promotes a meditative state.*

- **Sheetali Pranayama (Cooling Breath):** *Sheetali involves inhaling through a rolled tongue or pursed lips, creating a cooling sensation. Exhale through the nose. This technique reduces stress, lowers body temperature, and calms the mind.*

- **Kumbhaka (Breath Retention):** *Kumbhaka involves holding the breath after inhalation (Antara Kumbhaka) or after exhalation (Bahya Kumbhaka). This practice enhances lung capacity,* *increases awareness, and can have meditative benefits.*

Remember, these breathing techniques should be practiced with awareness and gradually. It's advisable to learn them under the guidance of a qualified yoga instructor to ensure proper execution and to address any individual concerns or limitations.

CHAPTER 4
BUILDING A CONSISTENCE PRACTICE

1.1 Creating Your Yoga Routine:

A regular yoga routine can contribute to physical and mental well-being by enhancing flexibility, strength, and balance, as well as promoting relaxation and stress reduction. It may also improve focus and mindfulness, fostering a holistic approach to health.
*Certainly! Creating a yoga routine for beginners involves careful consideration of various factors. **Here's a step-by-step guide:***

- ***Assessment of Fitness Level:** Begin by assessing the individual's current fitness level, flexibility, and any existing health conditions.*

- ***Define Goals:** Identify specific goals such as improving flexibility, reducing stress, or enhancing overall fitness. Tailor the routine to align with these objectives.*

- **Select Yoga Style:** Choose a beginner-friendly yoga style, such as Hatha or Vinyasa, which focuses on foundational poses and breath control.

- **Warm-Up:** Start with gentle warm-up exercises to prepare the body for yoga. Include light stretches and joint rotations to increase blood flow.

- **Basic Poses:** Introduce fundamental yoga poses like Mountain Pose, Downward-Facing Dog, and Warrior Poses. Emphasize proper alignment and encourage modifications for individual comfort.

- **Breathing Exercises (Pranayama):** Incorporate basic pranayama techniques like diaphragmatic breathing or ujjayi breath. Highlight the importance of mindful breathing throughout the routine.

- **Sequencing:***Organize the routine with a logical flow. Progress from easier poses to slightly more challenging ones, ensuring a gradual build-up.*

- **Duration:** *Keep the initial sessions shorter (around 20-30 minutes) to accommodate beginners' stamina. Gradually increase the duration as they become more comfortable.*

- **Balance and Flexibility:** *Include poses that improve balance and flexibility. These can include Tree Pose, Triangle Pose, and seated stretches.*

- **Cool Down:** *Conclude the routine with a cool-down segment, incorporating relaxing poses such as Child's Pose and Corpse Pose. This helps in reducing muscle tension.*

- **Mindfulness and Relaxation:** *Allocate time for mindfulness and relaxation. Guided meditation or Savasana (Corpse*

Pose) can be beneficial for mental well-being.

- ***Consistency and Progression:*** *Encourage regular practice and emphasize the importance of gradual progression. Advise participants to listen to their bodies and not push beyond their limits.*

- ***Educational Components:*** *Provide educational information about the benefits of each pose and how they contribute to overall well-being. This enhances participants' understanding and engagement.*

- ***Modifications:*** *Emphasize the importance of modifications to accommodate individual needs and limitations. Encourage the use of props like blocks and straps for added support.*

- ***Encouragement and Support:*** *Foster a supportive environment by offering positive reinforcement. Remind* *participants that yoga is a personal journey, and progress is achieved over time.*

- ***Feedback and Adjustment:*** *Gather feedback from participants to make necessary adjustments. This ensures the routine evolves to meet their changing needs and abilities.*

By following these steps, you can create a well-rounded and safe yoga routine tailored to the needs of beginners.

2.2 Overcoming Common Challenges:

Common challenges in yoga include maintaining consistency in practice, overcoming physical limitations or injuries, finding time for regular sessions in a busy schedule, dealing with distractions during practice, and mastering advanced poses. Additionally, some individuals may struggle with patience in seeing progress or face mental barriers such as self-doubt or comparison to others in the yoga community. It's essential to approach yoga with patience and a focus on personal growth. Here are step by step guide of overcoming this challenges :

- ***Set Realistic Goals:*** *Begin with achievable goals to build confidence. Setting realistic expectations helps avoid frustration and encourages a gradual progression in yoga practice.*

- ***Choose the Right Class:*** *Select a beginner-friendly class or instructor. Look for classes labeled "gentle" or "beginner" to ensure the pace and poses are suitable for newcomers.*

- ***Invest in Quality Equipment:*** *Purchase a good yoga mat and comfortable clothing to enhance your practice. Having the right equipment can improve stability and reduce discomfort during poses.*

- ***Learn Basic Poses:*** *Focus on fundamental poses like Mountain Pose, Downward Dog, and Child's Pose. Mastering these foundational postures* builds a strong base for more advanced poses.

- ***Practice Regularly:*** *Consistency is key. Establish a regular practice routine, even if it's just a few minutes each day. Regularity helps in building strength, flexibility, and overall improvement.*

- ***Listen to Your Body:*** *Pay attention to how your body feels during practice. Avoid pushing yourself too hard and modify poses as needed. Respect your body's limits to prevent injuries.*

- ***Breath Awareness:*** *Focus on your breath during practice. Learn proper breathing techniques like Ujjayi breath to enhance relaxation and concentration, promoting a mindful yoga experience.*

- ***Stay Patient and Positive:*** *Progress in yoga takes time. Embrace the learning process with patience and maintain a* *positive mindset. Celebrate small achievements along the way.*

- ***Use Props When Needed:*** *Props like blocks or straps can assist in maintaining proper alignment and ease into poses. Don't hesitate to incorporate props to enhance your practice.*

- ***Seek Guidance and Feedback:*** *Join a yoga community or seek guidance from experienced practitioners or instructors. Getting feedback helps correct form and ensures you're on the right track.*

- ***Warm-Up and Cool Down:*** *Always start with a gentle warm-up to prepare your body for the practice and end with a cool-down to relax muscles. This helps in preventing injuries and promoting flexibility.*

- ***Educate Yourself:****Learn about the philosophy and principles of yoga. Understanding the holistic approach of yoga beyond physical postures can* *deepen your appreciation for the practice.*

Remember, progress in yoga is a personal journey, and everyone's experience is unique.

CHAPTER 5
EXPLORING DIFFERENT YOGA STYLES

1.1 Overview of Popular Yoga Styles:

Yoga encompasses various styles, each with its unique focus and techniques. Some popular styles include:

- **Hatha Yoga:** Focuses on basic postures (asanas) and breath control (pranayama). Ideal for beginners to build a strong foundation.

- **Vinyasa Yoga:** Involves flowing from one pose to another in coordination with breath. Great for improving flexibility and building strength.

- **Iyengar Yoga:** Emphasizes precise alignment in postures with the help of props. Ideal for beginners wanting to understand correct form.

- ***Ashtanga Yoga:*** *Involves a set sequence of poses performed in a specific order, promoting strength, flexibility, and focus.*

- ***Bikram Yoga:*** *Consists of a series of 26 postures practiced in a heated room. The heat aids flexibility and detoxification.*

- ***Kundalini Yoga:*** *Focuses on awakening spiritual energy through a combination of postures, breathwork, and meditation.*

- ***Restorative Yoga:*** *Emphasizes relaxation and rejuvenation, using props to support the body in passive poses for extended periods.*

- ***Yin Yoga:*** *Involves holding poses for longer durations, targeting connective tissues.Excellent for increasing flexibility and promoting relaxation.*

Choose a style that aligns with your goals and preferences, and consider trying a few classes to find what resonates best with you.

2.2 Finding the Style That Fits You:

Finding the right yoga style is crucial for beginners as it helps create a positive and enjoyable experience. It ensures that the practice aligns with your preferences, fitness level, and goals, making it more sustainable. This tailored approach enhances motivation, promotes consistency, and contributes to a fulfilling journey in exploring the benefits of yoga. Here are major process of findind the right style that fits your body :

- *Explore Different Styles: Begin by exploring various yoga styles like Hatha, Vinyasa, Ashtanga, and more. Each style has its unique characteristics and pace, allowing you to find one that resonates with you.*

- *Consider Physical Abilities: Assess your physical abilities and any health considerations. Some styles are more vigorous, while others focus on gentle movements. Choose a style that aligns with your current fitness level and health conditions.*

- ***Understand Your Goals:*** *Define your yoga goals. Whether you seek relaxation, flexibility, strength, or a combination, different styles emphasize various aspects. For example, if stress relief is a priority, you might lean towards restorative or yin yoga.*

- ***Attend Beginner Classes:*** *Attend beginner-friendly classes for different styles. Many studios offer introductory sessions, allowing you to experience the basics of each style. This hands-on approach helps you gauge your comfort and enjoyment.*

- ***Explore Online Resources:*** *Utilize online resources like videos and articles to deepen your understanding of each style. Follow guided practices and observe how your body responds to different movements and sequences.*

- ***Listen to Your Body:*** *Pay attention to how your body feels during and after each session. If you enjoy the practice and feel invigorated or relaxed, it's a positive sign that the style may be a good fit for you.*

- ***Experiment with Instructors:*** *Different instructors bring their unique teaching styles to each practice. Attend classes with various instructors within the chosen style to find someone whose guidance resonates with you.*

- ***Consistency is Key:*** *Give each style a fair chance by consistently practicing it for a few sessions. Sometimes, it takes time to fully appreciate the benefits and nuances of a particular yoga style.*

- ***Reflect on Preferences:*** *Reflect on your preferences. Do you enjoy a more structured and disciplined practice, or do you prefer a free-flowing and creative* *approach? Your personal preferences play a crucial role in finding the right style for you.*

- ***Combine Elements:*** *Don't hesitate to combine elements from different styles. Yoga is a versatile practice, and you can customize your routine to include aspects from various traditions, creating a practice that uniquely suits you.*

Remember, finding the right yoga style is a personal journey. It's about discovering what resonates with your body, mind, and spirit. Enjoy the exploration and allow yourself the flexibility to evolve in your practice.

CHAPTER 6
INTEGRATING YOGA INTO DAILY LIFE

1.1 Bringing Yoga Off the Mat:

"Bringing yoga off the mat" refers to applying the principles and mindfulness cultivated during yoga practice to daily life. It involves integrating the physical, mental, and spiritual aspects of yoga into one's actions, attitudes, and interactions beyond the yoga studio or mat. It encourages a holistic approach to well-being and mindfulness in various aspects of life. Here are the step by step guide 2 achieving this:

- *Mindful Awareness: Begin by cultivating mindfulness in everyday activities. Pay attention to your breath, sensations, and surroundings, fostering a present-moment awareness.*

- *Intention Setting: Establish clear intentions for your day, aligning them with yogic principles such as compassion, gratitude, and self-awareness. This sets a positive tone for your actions.*

- ***Yamas and Niyamas:*** *Explore the ethical guidelines of yoga, known as Yamas (restraints) and Niyamas (observances). Apply principles like non-violence, truthfulness, contentment, and self-discipline in interactions and decision-making.*

- ***Asana Practice Beyond the Mat:*** *Extend yoga poses into daily movements. Focus on alignment and breath during routine tasks like standing, walking, or sitting, promoting physical awareness and well-being.*

- ***Breath Awareness:*** *Integrate pranayama (breath control) techniques into daily life. Practice conscious breathing during stressful situations or mundane activities, promoting a sense of calm and mental clarity.*

- ***Mindful Eating:*** *Apply yogic principles to your diet by cultivating awareness during meals. Eat mindfully, savoring each bite, and choose foods that nourish your body and mind.*

- ***Seva (Selfless Service):*** *Incorporate seva into your life, embracing the concept of selfless service. Volunteer or support others without expecting anything in return, fostering a sense of community and compassion.*

- ***Mind-Body Connection:*** *Emphasize the mind-body connection beyond yoga poses. Recognize how thoughts and emotions affect physical sensations, and vice versa, promoting holistic well-being.*

- ***Mindfulness in Relationships:*** *Bring yoga off the mat by applying its principles to relationships. Practice empathy, active listening, and open communication, fostering harmonious connections with others.*

- ***Reflection and Self-Inquiry:*** *Dedicate time for self-reflection and introspection. Journaling or meditation can help you understand your thoughts and emotions, supporting personal growth and self-discovery.*

- ***Gratitude Practice:*** *Cultivate gratitude by acknowledging and appreciating positive aspects of your life. Regularly express gratitude, whether internally or through gestures, to foster a positive mindset.*

- ***Continuous Learning:*** *Embrace a mindset of continuous learning and self-improvement. Explore new aspects of yoga philosophy, attend workshops, or read literature that expands your understanding of yoga beyond the physical practice.*

By incorporating these steps, you can bring the essence of yoga off the mat and weave its transformative principles into the fabric of your daily life.

2.2 Sustaining a Lifelong Yoga Habit

Sustaining a lifelong yoga habit involves regular practice, adapting to your evolving needs, embracing a holistic approach, and finding joy in the journey rather than focusing solely on achievements. It's about creating a sustainable, balanced routine that aligns with your lifestyle. This can be achieved through these step by step guide :

- *Set Clear Intentions: Define why you want to practice yoga for a lifetime. Whether it's for physical fitness, mental well-being, or spiritual growth, having a clear intention will help you stay committed.*

- *Start Slow and Gradual: Begin with beginner-friendly yoga poses and routines. Avoid pushing yourself too hard initially to prevent burnout or injuries.*

- ***Consistency is Key:*** *Establish a consistent practice schedule. Even short sessions regularly can be more beneficial than sporadic, longer sessions.*

- ***Explore Different Styles:*** *Experiment with various styles of yoga to find what resonates with you. There are styles like Hatha, Vinyasa, or Kundalini, each offering unique benefits.*

- ***Build a Routine:*** *Incorporate yoga into your daily routine. This could be a morning or evening ritual, making it easier to integrate seamlessly into your lifestyle.*

- ***Use Online Resources:*** *Leverage online platforms for guided sessions. There are many apps and websites providing classes for all levels, allowing you to practice anywhere, anytime.*

- ***Attend Classes:*** *Join local yoga classes or workshops. The guidance of an* instructor can help refine your practice, ensuring proper form and technique.

- **Invest in Quality Equipment:** *Purchase a comfortable yoga mat and other props to enhance your practice. Having the right equipment can make your sessions more enjoyable and effective.*

- **Listen to Your Body:** *Pay attention to your body's signals. If you feel discomfort or pain, modify or skip poses. Adapt your practice to suit your individual needs and abilities.*

- **Mindfulness and Breathwork:** *Incorporate mindfulness and breathwork (pranayama) into your routine. These aspects are integral to yoga and contribute significantly to overall well-being.*

- **Set Realistic Goals:** *Establish achievable milestones. Whether it's holding a specific pose or increasing flexibility,* *setting realistic goals can motivate you to progress without feeling overwhelmed.*

- ***Connect with a Community:*** *Join a yoga community, either in-person or online. Sharing experiences and challenges with others can provide motivation and a sense of belonging.*

- ***Educate Yourself:*** *Learn about the philosophy and principles of yoga. Understanding the broader context can deepen your appreciation and commitment to the practice.*

- ***Adapt to Life Changes:*** *Be flexible in adapting your practice to life changes. Whether it's a busy schedule or physical limitations, find ways to modify your routine to suit your current circumstances.*

- ***Celebrate Progress:*** *Acknowledge and celebrate your achievements along the way. Whether it's mastering a* *challenging pose or consistently sticking to your routine, recognizing progress reinforces your commitment.*

By incorporating these steps, beginners can gradually cultivate and sustain a lifelong yoga habit that contributes to their overall well-being.